Ketogenic Cocktails

The Ultimate Delicious and Keto Friendly Cocktails for Beginners to Stay Lean and Enjoy the Process

Jenny Kern

Table Of Contents

Introduction

Thank you for purchasing this book. Drinkers appreciate and go in search of more refined ingredients, the balance and balance of flavors and aromas, just like sommeliers do to choose a wine suitable for the occasion; in fact, with always new and numerous recipes designed for specific moments, which in addition to the classic between meals meet the combination with food and also the daytime hours of the day, cocktails have invaded our days, dinners, lunches, brunches independently from their more or less alcohol content. I hope you enjoy my keto cocktails and entice you to become a true expert in this art.

Enjoy.

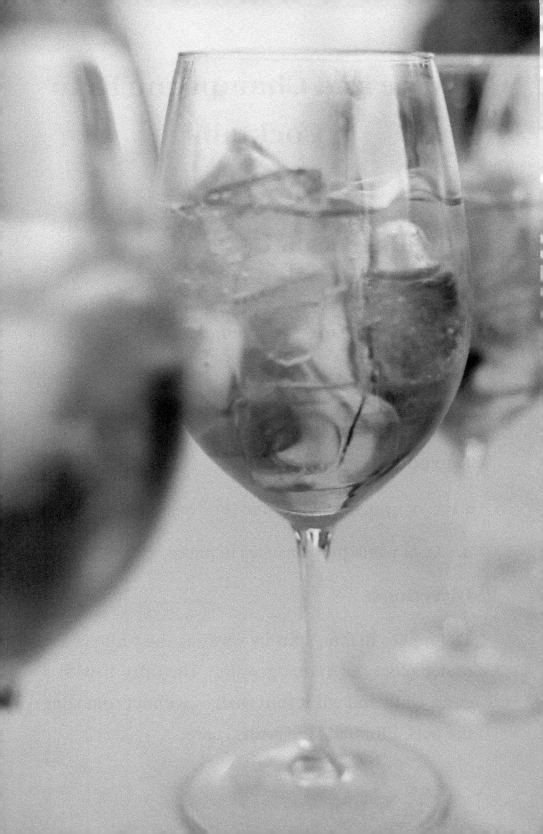

Wine and Champagne Keto Cocktails

Bellini cocktail

Preparation time: 20 minutes

Servings: 2

Ingredients:

1.1oz. of brut sparkling wine (or Prosecco)

4.4oz. of white pulp peaches in puree

Directions:

To prepare Bellini, start by washing the white peach under plenty of running water. Then dry it with a clean cloth and cut it into wedges without removing the peel. Eliminate the central core.

Add the peach to a mixer and whisk until the puree is obtained. Now filter the peach puree with a narrow mesh strainer placed on top of a bowl.

You will need to obtain a homogeneous pulp. Pour it into a shaker and add the very cold Brut sparkling wine. Briefly mix the ingredients with a stirrer (the long-handled spoon used for making cocktails).

Apply the strainer, i.e. the special shaker strainer, over the shaker and filter the cocktail directly into the flutes. Serve your Bellini.

Tips:

Bellini Cocktail should be consumed as soon as it is ready.

Rossini

Preparation time: 50 minutes

Servings: 3

Ingredients:

1 bottle of cold Prosecco or champagne

White wine to taste

Lemon juice to taste

2.5oz. of strawberries

1 teaspoon of sugar

Directions:

Clean the strawberries.

Drain them, cut them into slices or cubes, and let them macerate for 30 minutes with 1 teaspoon of sugar and a few drops of lemon.

Blend the strawberries, pour them into a glass bowl. Slowly add a bottle of cold Prosecco or champagne.

The cocktail is ready, mix gently and serve.

Tips:

Accompany this cocktail with cheese and rosemary pretzels or sandwiches and puff pastries.

Rosé Frosé

Preparation time: 5 minutes

Servings: 2

Ingredients:

2 oz pomegranate vodka

1 cup rosé wine

2 oz pink grapefruit juice

½ oz fresh lemon juice

½ oz - 1 oz simple syrup

1 ¼ cup crushed ice

Directions:

Add vodka, wine, grapefruit juice, lemon juice, and simple syrup in a blender, blend for a few seconds to combine.

Add ice to the blender and blend until smooth.

Pour into a chilled cocktail glass and garnish with a slice of pink grapefruit.

Limoncello Champagne

Preparation time: 10 minutes

Servings: 8

Ingredients:

8 tbsps. limoncello, or liquor with lemon flavor

8 lemon rind strips

1 750-ml. bottle chilled Brut champagne

4 tsp. fresh lemon juice

Directions:

Roll each strip of the lemon rind up then place each one into a champagne flute.

Add one tablespoon of the liquor and a half teaspoon of the juice to every glass.

Pour the champagne evenly among the glasses. Serve right away.

Cranberry Champagne Cocktail

Preparation time: 10 minutes

Servings: 7

Ingredients:

3 tbsps. sugar

¼ c. water

½ c. whole berry cranberry sauce

4 c. dry prosecco, chilled

¾ c. vodka

Directions:

Mix sugar and one-fourth cup water in a pan. Set the pan over medium heat. Cook this mixture for around five minutes or until you notice that the sugar has melted. Remove the pan from heat.

Pour in the cranberry juice then let the mixture sit to cool. Add the vodka then pour the mixture into a bowl. Cover the bowl and store the drink in your fridge for up to four hours.

Use a sieve lined with cheesecloth to strain the mixture into a jar. Discard any solids. Make sure that the jar has an airtight lid to secure the mixture. Chill it until it is ready to use.

Spoon around two tablespoons of cranberry juice into one champagne flute. Top it with wine. Serve.

Lemon Sparkling Cocktail

Preparation time: 10 minutes

Servings: 8

Ingredients:

2 2/3 c. champagne

½ c. lemonade concentrate, frozen then thawed

1 c. gin, chilled

Optional Ingredient: tarragon sprigs

Directions:

Mix the lemonade concentrate and the gin in a pitcher. Let it chill until you are ready to serve.

Before serving, pour champagne into the mixture. Gently stir. Add tarragon sprigs as garnishing, if you are planning to use them. Serve.

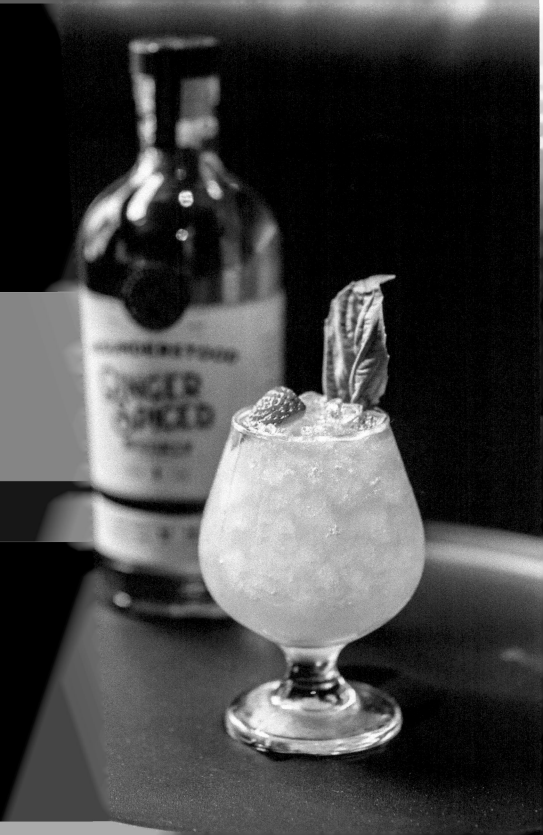

Gin Keto Cocktails

Gin Impact

Preparation time: 10 minutes

Servings: 2

Ingredients:

22 milliliters freshly squeezed lemon juice

22 milliliters sugar syrup

1 dash bitters

60 milliliters chilled water

60 milliliters London dry gin

Directions:

Shake ingredients with ice and strain into ice-filled glass. Garnish using lemon slices.

Pink Grapefruit Punch

Preparation time: 10 minutes

Servings: 2

Ingredients:

100 ml (3.4 oz.) gin

200 ml (6.8 oz.) pink grapefruit juice

50 ml (1.7 oz.) Campari

750 ml (25.4 oz.) rose wine

25 ml (0.85 oz.) red vermouth

½ bunch of thyme

1 tbsp honey

Ice cubes

Directions:

Pour all the ingredients into a punch bowl.

Add ice and stir gently.

Garnish with thyme.

Spiced Apple Snaps Fizz

Preparation time: 10 minutes

Servings: 2

Ingredients:

200 ml (6.8 oz.) bottle sparkling wine

50 ml (1.7 oz.) gin

4 tbsp apple juice

The juice of 1 lemon

Ice cubes

Ground cinnamon

½ small apple, thinly sliced

Directions:

Pour the gin into a cocktail shaker.

Add the apple and lemon juices, some cinnamon, and ice. Shake well.

Pour into 2 fluted glasses.

Add the sparkling wine.

Top up with additional cinnamon and garnish with the apple slices.

Blackberry Ginger Gin

Preparation time: 10 minutes

Servings: 2

Ingredients:

Gin (1, 750ml bottle)

Blackberries (6 oz)

Ginger (1/2 cup, sliced, peeled)

Directions:

Combine all the ingredients in a glass airtight container. Seal and shake a few times to mix the infusion.

Store for approximately 9 days in a cool, dark, and secure place. Ensuring to taste it daily, as well as to shake it to release more flavor.

For a lesser taste of ginger, add the ginger 3 days after the blackberries.

When the flavor is to your liking, strain out the solids and rebottle the gin.

Serve over ice or in a tonic. Enjoy!

Cucumber Rose Gin

Preparation time: 15 minutes

Servings: 12

Ingredients:

Gin (1, (750 ml) bottle)

Cucumber (1, sliced)

Rose buds (1/2 oz, dried)

Directions:

In a medium-sized mason jar place all the ingredients.

Seal and shake a few times to agitate the infusion.

Store in a cool, dry place and shake for approximately 1 to 3 times each day. Also taste daily to check on flavor.

Next, strain through cheesecloth when at the desired flavor. Rebottle the infused booze and store it in the refrigerator.

Serve over ice or in a tonic. A rose bud makes a pretty garnish.

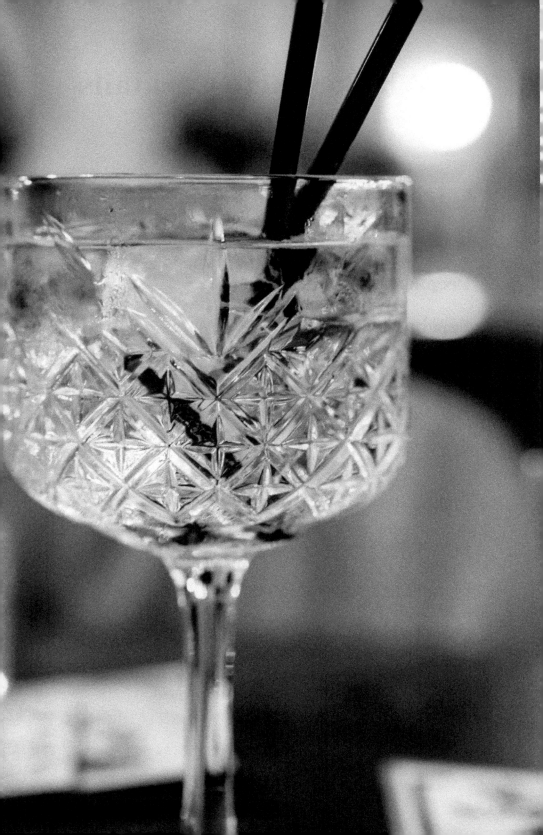

Whiskey Keto Cocktails

Iron Mountain

Preparation time: 10 minutes

Servings: 2

Ingredients:

½ fresh egg white

15 milliliters dry vermouth

15 milliliters lemon juice

15 milliliters sweet vermouth

45 milliliters bourbon whiskey

Directions:

Shake ingredients with ice and strain into chilled glass. Garnish using maraschino cherry.

Irish coffee

Preparation time: 10 minutes

Servings: 2

Ingredients:

15 milliliters muscovado sugar syrup

1⅓ oz. whipping cream

45 milliliters Irish whiskey

2½ oz. hot filter coffee

Directions:

Warm a heat-proof glass. Lightly whip cream. Pour whiskey, sugar syrup, and hot coffee into warmed glass until it is about three-quarters full and stir. Float whipped cream by pouring over the back of a warmed spoon.

Tipperary

Preparation time: 10 minutes

Servings: 1

Ingredients:

3/4 oz. Irish whiskey

3/4 oz. Chartreuse

3/4 oz. sweet vermouth

3 or 4 ice cubes

Directions:

In a mixing glass, mix all ingredients and stir well. Transfer into a cocktail glass through a strainer.

Classic Sazerac

Preparation time: 10 minutes

Servings: 10

Ingredients:

50ml sugar syrup

1 tsp Peychaud's bitters

0.5 tsp Angostura bitters

200ml whiskey, the rye variety works well with this cocktail

2 tsp absinthe

25ml cold water

A handful of ice cubes

A little orange zest to decorate

Directions:

Take four whiskey tumblers and add the absinthe to just one glass, swirling around the bottom of the glass

Pour the absinthe into the next glass and repeat, covering all four glasses

Take a large mixing jug and add the bitters, the whiskey, and the sugar syrup. Add the water and ice cubes. Combine until he outside of the jug feels icy

Use a strainer to pour the cocktail into each glass equally

Take a piece of orange zest and twist it over one glass, dropping it inside. Repeat with all four glasses

Refreshing Mint Julep

Preparation time: 5 minutes

Servings: 1

Ingredients:

65ml bourbon

12.5ml sugar syrup

10 fresh mint leaves

A handful of ice cubes

Crushed ice

Directions:

Take a cocktail shaker and add the bourbon, sugar syrup, and mint. Add the ice cubes and shake well

Fill a julep glass or a highball glass with crushed ice

Use a strainer to pour the cocktail into the glass

Use a long-handled spoon and churn the cocktail by moving it around quickly inside the glass

Add a little more crushed ice and serve with a straw

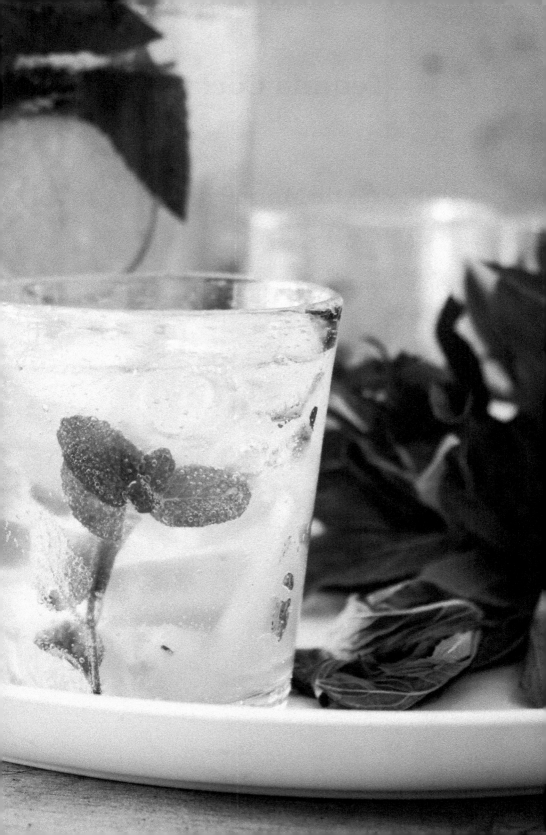

Tequila Cocktails

A Fantastic Margarita

Preparation time: 10 minutes

Servings: 2

Ingredients:

2 cups limeade prepared from concentrate

1/2 cup pineapple juice

1/2 cup orange juice

2 fluid ounces tequila

1 fluid ounce orange liqueur

Directions:

Salt the rims of 2 large margarita glasses. To do so, pour salt onto a small plate, moisten the rims of the glasses on a damp towel and press them into the salt.

In a pitcher combine limeade, pineapple juice, orange juice, tequila, and orange liqueur. Stir well and pour into the glasses, being careful not to rinse off the salt.

Perfect Margarita

Preparation time: 10 minutes

Servings: 2

Ingredients:

1 fluid ounce premium tequila

3/4 fluid ounce brandy-based orange liqueur (such as Grand Marnier®)

3/4 fluid ounce Cointreau

3/4 fluid ounce simple syrup

1 fluid ounce raspberry-flavored liqueur

1 lime, juiced

1/2 cup sweet and sour mix

Directions:

Salt the rims of 2 large margarita glasses. To do so, pour salt onto a small plate, moisten the rims of the glasses on a damp towel and press them into the salt.

In a cocktail mixer 3/4 full of ice, combine tequila, Grand Marnier, Cointreau, simple syrup, raspberry liqueur, and lime juice. Pour in sweet and sour until ice is covered. Shake vigorously and strain into glass.

Kerman

Preparation time: 10 minutes

Servings: 2

Ingredients:

1½ oz. silver tequila

¾ oz. pistachio syrup

¾ oz. lime juice

Pink salt

Ice

Directions:

Salt the rim of the glass

Pour ¾ oz. of lime juice, ¾ oz. of pistachio syrup, and 1½ oz. of silver tequila into a shaker

Fill the shaker with ice cubes and shake gently then strain

Cancun Martini

Preparation time: 10 minutes

Servings: 2

Ingredients:

1 (1.5 fluid ounce) jigger tequila (such as Jose Cuervo®)

1/2 fluid ounce coffee-flavored liqueur (such as Trader Vic's®)

1 maraschino cherry

Directions:

Pour tequila and coffee-flavored liqueur into a shaker filled with ice; cover and shake until chilled. Strain drink into a martini glass. Garnish with a maraschino cherry.

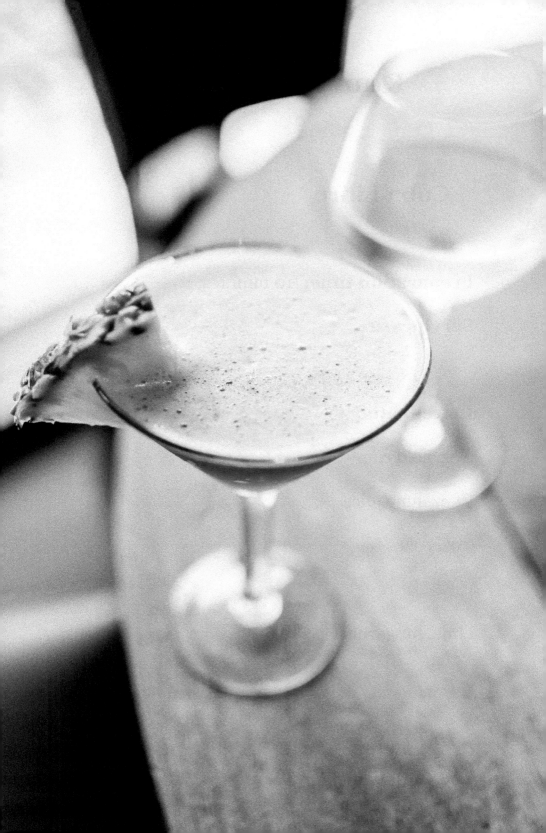

Rum Keto Cocktails

Cuba Libre

Preparation time: 10 minutes

Servings: 2

Ingredients:

2 oz. gold rum

½ oz. lime juice

5 oz. cola

Ice

Lime, for garnish

Directions:

Fill a highball glass to the top with ice

Pour in ½ oz. of lime juice and 2 oz. of gold rum

Top up with cola and stir gently

Garnish with 2 lime wheels

The Iconic Pina Colada

Preparation time: 10 minutes

Servings: 2

Ingredients:

60ml white rum

120ml fresh pineapple juice

60ml coconut cream

A handful of ice cubes

A slice of pineapple for decoration

Directions:

Take a regular blender and add all the ingredients, except for the decorative pineapple

Blitz the mixture until a smooth consistency occurs

Take a tall cocktail glass and pour the mixture inside

Add the slice of pineapple as decoration

Minty Mojito

Preparation time: 10 minutes

Servings: 2

Ingredients:

60ml white rum

1 tsp sugar

A little soda water, according to your taste

The juice of 1 lime

A few fresh mint leaves

A handful of ice cubes

Directions:

Take a small jug and add the sugar, mint leaves (leave a few to one side for decoration), and the lime juice

Use a muddler to combine, carefully crushing the leaves

Take a tall cocktail glass and add the muddled mixture into the bottom

Add a handful of ice cubes on top

Carefully pour the rum into the glass

Take a long bar spoon and stir carefully to combine the ingredients

Add a little soda water on top

Decorate with the other mint leaves

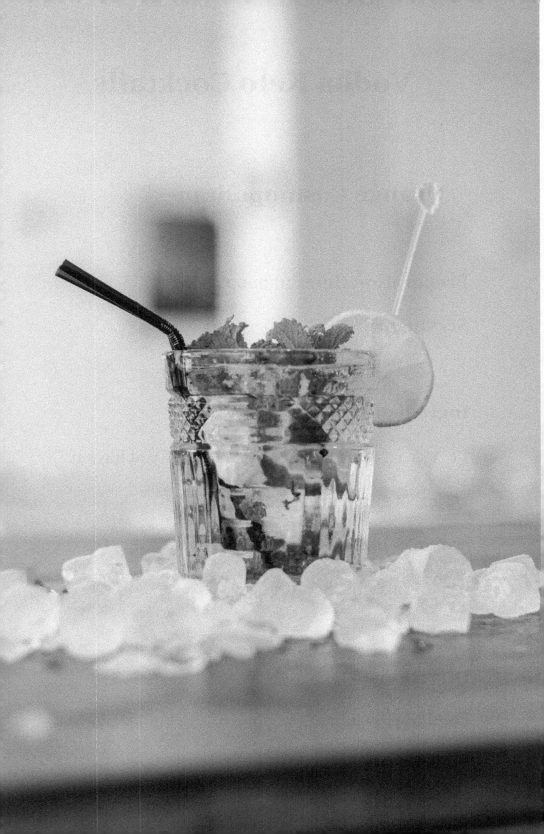

Vodka Keto Cocktails

Orange Cosmopolitan

Preparation time: 10 minutes

Servings: 3

Ingredients:

1 & 1/2 oz. of vodka, Absolut Citron if you have it

1/2 oz. of cranberry juice

3/4 oz. of lime, fresh

3/4 oz. of Triple Sec, orange

Directions:

Combine the ingredients in a tin cocktail shaker.

Add filtered ice.

Vigorously shake, till tin has frosted fully over.

Strain liquid into a pre-chilled cocktail or highball glass.

Use lime twist for garnishing. Serve.

Chocolate Martini

Preparation time: 10 minutes

Servings: 3

Ingredients:

2 oz vodka

1 1/2 oz crème de cacao, white Hershey Hug or Kiss for garnish powdered cocoa for rimming

Directions:

Pour the ingredients into a shaker with ice cubes.

Shake vigorously.

Strain into a chilled cocktail glass rimmed with cocoa.

Chilled Cosmopolitan

Preparation time: 10 minutes

Servings: 3

Ingredients:

1 1/2 oz vodka

1 oz Cointreau

1/2 oz fresh lime juice 1/4 oz cranberry juice orange peel for garnish

Directions:

Shake all the ingredients with ice in a cocktail shaker.

Strain into a chilled cocktail glass.

Garnish with an orange peel.

Diamond Martini

Preparation time: 10 minutes

Servings: 4

Ingredients:

Dash of premium dry vermouth 1/2 cup premium grain vodka, frozen lemon wedge

Directions:

Chill a cocktail glass.

Pour the dry vermouth and vodka into the glass.

Twist the lemon wedge over the drink.

Run the lemon wedge around the rim of the glass.

Flirtini

Preparation time: 10 minutes

Servings: 3

Ingredients:

2 pieces fresh pineapple

1/2 oz Cointreau

1/2 oz vodka

1 oz pineapple juice 3 oz Champagne maraschino cherry for garnish

Directions:

Muddle the pineapple pieces and Cointreau in the bottom of a mixing glass.

Add the vodka and pineapple juice.

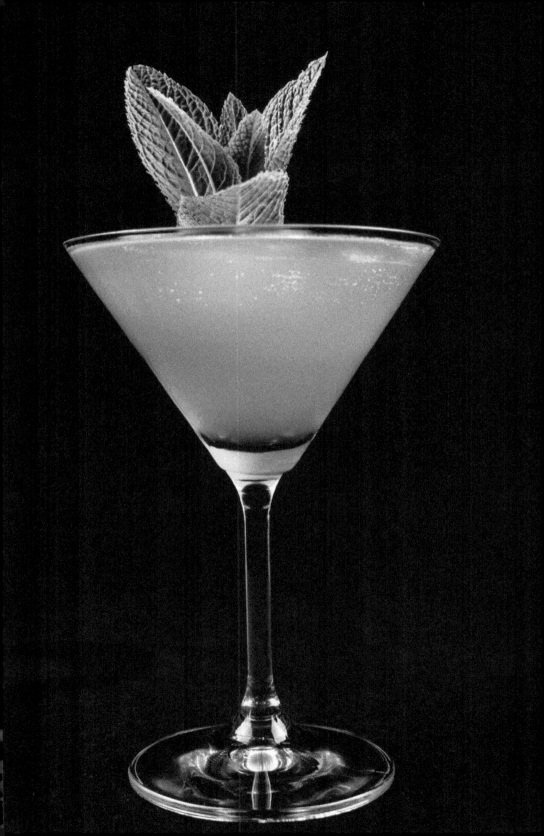

Keto Liqueurs

Blow Job

Preparation time: 10 minutes

Servings: 2

Ingredients:

½ ounces anisette liqueur

½ ounces Bailey's Irish cream

Whipped cream to garnish

Directions:

Measure the anisette into a jigger. Carefully pour into a chilled shot glass.

Measure the Bailey's into a jigger. Slowly pour the Bailey's over the back of the spoon allowing it to pool on top of the anisette.

Garnish with whipped cream.

Mocha Maria Recipe

Preparation time: 10 minutes

Servings: 2

Ingredients:

Tia Maria® coffee liqueur (2 oz)

Creme de cacao (2 oz, dark)

Irish cream (2 oz)

Directions:

In a cocktail shaker half-filled with ice add ingredients and shake.

When finished, pour over ice in a highball glass.

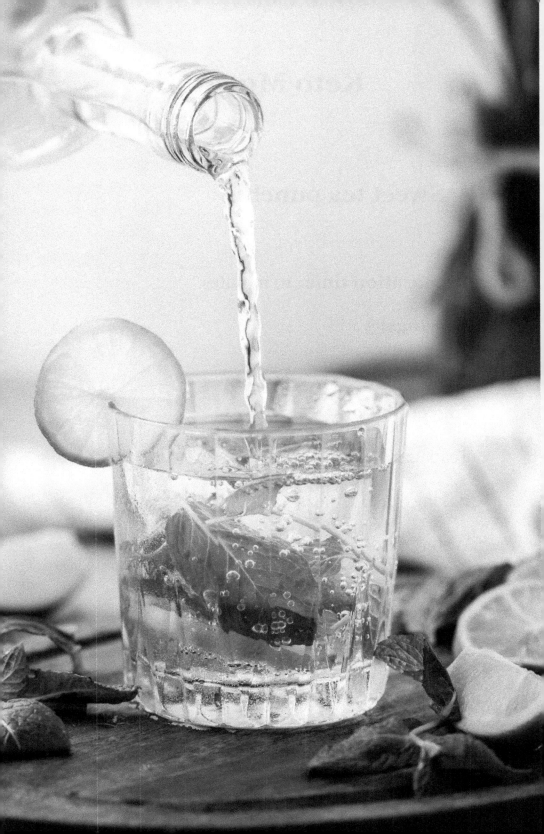

Keto Mocktails

Sweet tea punch

Preparation time: 10 minutes

Servings: 3

Ingredients:

Teabag: 1

Baking Soda: 1/8 oz.

Water: 6 oz.

Maple Syrup: 2 oz.

Ice as required

Directions:

Take the teabag and add it to a saucepan.

Add the baking soda to the pan.

Add in water and boil everything.

Remove the teabag and let it cool for some time.

Put ice in the serving glass and pour the tea in it.

Mix with the maple syrup and serve.

Chocolate Mocktails

Preparation time: 10 minutes

Servings: 4

Ingredients:

½ of a Cup of sugar

2 level Tbsp of natural cocoa powder

¼ of a tsp of ground cinnamon

1 Cup of water

2 Cups of almond milk

Lemon

1 Cup of ice.

Directions:

Take your lemon & cut it into wedges.

Put the sugar and cocoa powder into your bowl.

Stir the mixture until thoroughly combined.

Take two Tbsp of the mixture and transfer to a small plate.

Put the remainder of the mixture along with the cinnamon and water into your saucepan.

Place over medium-high heat & cook.

Whisk the mixture until the sugar has dissolved completely.

Using your knife, cut into the lemon wedge.

Take the wedge and run it around the rooms of the glasses.

Turn the glasses upside down and place them into the sugar.

Now take the syrup mixture and pour half of it into the cocktail shaker.

Add a cup of ice & a cup of almond milk.

Apply to cover the shaker and shake until the drink has chilled.

Divide the drink between the glasses.

Use the same process for the remaining two glasses.

Non-Alcoholic Sangria

Preparation time: 10 minutes

Servings: 3

Ingredients:

2 Cups of boiling water

2 black teabags or 2 tsp of loose-leaf tea in an infuser

2 cinnamon sticks

½ of a Cup of sugar

3 Cups of pomegranate juice

1 Cup of freshly squeezed orange juice

1 orange, sliced into thin rounds

1 lemon

1 lime

1 apple

3 Cups of carbonated water

Directions:

Begin by cutting the lemon in the lime into rounds.

Take the apple and remove the core.

Now cut into half-inch chunks.

Put the water into the saucepan and place it over medium heat.

Bring the water to a boil.

Take the teabags and cinnamon sticks and put them into your bowl.

Pour the water into the bowl & steep for about five minutes.

Take out the teabags and toss.

Add the sugar and stir until completely dissolved.

Take the tea, pomegranate juice, cinnamon sticks, orange, orange juice, lemon, apple, lime and place them in your jar or pitcher.

Placing the fridge for an hour or overnight.

Before serving add in the carbonated water.

This drink should be served over ice.

Sparkling Rosemary Limeade

Preparation time: 10 minutes

Servings: 3

Ingredients:

1 Cup of lime juice

¾ of a Cup of sugar

Peel of 2 limes

Two 4-inch sprigs of fresh rosemary, plus more to serve

4 to 6 Cups of chilled sparkling water

Directions:

Using your knife, or peeler, remove the peel from the limes.

Place the peels into a bowl for later use.

You can use either bottle lime juice or freshly squeezed.

Should you use freshly squeezed it requires approximately 6 limes.

Put the lime juice and the sugar into your saucepan.

Place the pan over medium and allow to simmer.

Reduce the heat and continue to cook until sugar has dissolved.

Be sure to stir often.

Now add the lime peel & Rosemary sprigs.

Continue to simmer for about a minute.

Turn the heat off.

Place a cover on the pan and place it in the fridge overnight.

Pour the mixture through the strainer.

Remove the peel along with the Rosemary.

Take the liquid mixture and combine it with sparkling water.

Transfer to a jar or bottle.

This drink should be served over ice using a sprig of Rosemary as garnish.

Asian Pear Sparkler

Preparation time: 10 minutes

Servings: 3

Ingredients:

1 Cup of freshly pressed Asian pear juice

1 tsp of lemon juice

¾ of a Cup of honey

¼ of a Cup of sugar

1 4-inch sprig of fresh rosemary

1 1-inch piece of fresh ginger, peeled and cut into coins

Small grating of fresh nutmeg

Ice

Soda water

Directions:

Begin by peeling the ginger.

Cut into shapes similar to small coins.

Take the pear juice, lemon juice, sugar, honey, ginger, Rosemary & nutmeg and put them into your saucepan.

Place over medium heat and bring to a boil.

Reduce the heat and allow the mixture to simmer for about five minutes.

Stir the mixture continuously while the sugar dissolves.

Now take the pan off the seed and set it to the side for about a half-hour.

Run this mixture through the strainer and toss the solids.

Allow the mixture to cool completely.

Fill your glass with ice halfway.

Put 3 Tbsp of syrup into the glass.

Finish filling with soda water.

Stir.

Elderberry Shrub

Preparation time: 10 minutes

Servings: 3

Ingredients:

1 Cup of elderberries

1 Cup of vinegar

About 1 & ½ Cups of sugar

Soda water to serve

Directions:

Place the elderberries into the colander.

Hold under running water until clean.

Transfer the berries to the jar & mash with a fork.

Now add vinegar to the jar and stir.

Apply lid to the jar and place in the fridge until the next day.

Periodically shake the jar or stir.

After removing the jar from the fridge, shake or stir.

Strain mixture and toss solids.

Measure the liquid and place it into the saucepan.

Add one cup of sugar for every cup of liquid.

Place the pan over medium-low heat.

Allow the mixture to reach a boil, stirring until the sugar has dissolved.

Continue to boil for five minutes.

Take off of the heat.

Set the pan aside to cool.

Transfer the mixture to a bottle and place it in the fridge.

Use one part of the mixture to six parts sparkling water one serving.

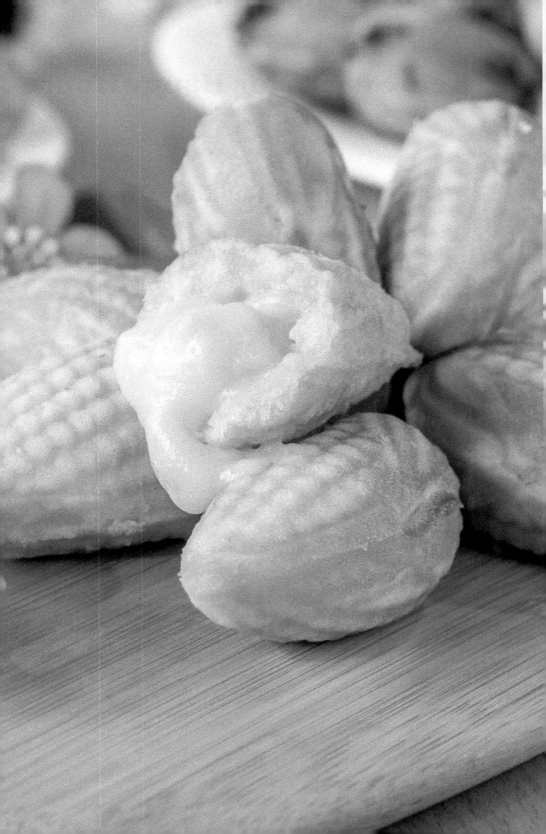

Keto Snacks for Happy Hour

Taco Flavored Cheddar Crisps

Preparation time: 5 minutes

Cooking Time: 10 minutes

Servings: 6 servings

Ingredients:

¾ c sharp cheddar cheese, finely shredded

¼ c parmesan cheese, finely shredded

¼ t chili powder

¼ t ground cumin

Directions:

Preheat the oven to 400 degrees.

Line cookie sheet with parchment paper

In a bowl, toss all ingredients together until well mixed.

Make 12 piles of cheese parchment paper.

Press down the cheese into a thin layer of cheese.

Bake for 5 minutes until the cheese is bubbly.

Let it cool on parchment paper.

When completely cool, peel the paper away from the crisps.

These are a good Keto substitute for chips. They are cheesy and crisp. Enjoy!

Nutrition: calories 198, fat 12, fiber 2, carbs 2, protein 35

Keto Seed Crispy Crackers

Preparation time: 10 minutes

Cooking Time: 45 minutes

Servings: 30 servings of 1 cracker

Ingredients:

⅓ cup almond flour

⅓ cup sunflower seed kernels

⅓ cup pumpkin seed kernels

⅓ cup flaxseed

⅓ cup chia seeds

1 tbsp. ground psyllium husk powder

1 tsp. salt

¼ cup melted coconut oil.

1 cup boiling water.

Directions:

Preheat the oven to 300 degrees.

Stir all dry ingredients together in a medium-sized bowl until thoroughly mixed.

Add coconut oil and boiling water to dry ingredients and stir until all ingredients are mixed well.

On a flat surface, roll the dough between two pieces of parchment paper until approximately ⅛ inch thick.

Slide the dough, still between parchment papers onto a baking sheet.

Remove the top layer of parchment paper and place dough on a baking sheet into the oven.

Bake for 40 minutes until golden brown.

Score the top of the dough into cracker-sized pieces.

Leave in the oven to cool down.

When the big cracker is cool, break into pieces.

These crackers can be stored in an airtight container after they are completely cool.

Nutrition: calories 340, fat 23, fiber 2, carbs 8, protein 28

Garlic Roasted Potatoes

Preparation time: 15 minutes

Cooking Time: 30 minutes

Servings: 4-6

Ingredients:

5 tbsp. vegetable oil

5 cloves garlic

2 lbs. baby potatoes

1 rosemary spring

½ cup stock

Salt and ground black pepper to taste

Directions:

Select the SAUTÉ setting on the Instant Pot and heat the oil. Add the garlic, potatoes, and rosemary. Cook, stirring occasionally, for 10 minutes or until the potatoes start to brown.

Using a fork, pierce the middle of each potato. Pour in the stock. Season with salt and pepper. Stir well. Press the CANCEL key to stop the SAUTÉ function.

Close and lock the lid. Select MANUAL and cook at HIGH pressure for 7 minutes. When the timer beeps, use a Quick Release. Carefully unlock the lid. Serve.

Nutrition: calories 340, fat 23, fiber 2, carbs 8, protein 28

Autumn Potatoes Salad

Preparation time: 10 minutes

Cooking Time: 25 minutes

Servings: 4-6

Ingredients:

1½ cups water

4 eggs

6 medium potatoes, peeled and cut into 1½ inch cubes

1 tbsp. dill pickle juice

1 cup homemade mayonnaise

2 tbsp. parsley, finely chopped

¼ cup onion, finely chopped

1 tbsp. mustard

Salt and ground black pepper to taste

Directions:

Pour the water into the Instant Pot and insert a steamer basket. Place the eggs and potatoes in the basket. Select MANUAL and cook at HIGH pressure for 5 minutes.

When the timer goes off, use a Quick Release. Carefully open the lid. Transfer the eggs to the bowl of cold water. Wait 2-3 minutes.

In another bowl, combine the dill pickle juice, mayo, parsley, onion, and mustard. Mix well. Add the potatoes and gently stir to coat with the sauce. Peel eggs, chop, and add to the salad. Stir well.

Season with salt and pepper, stir, and serve.

Nutrition: calories 270, fat 18, fiber 1, carbs 3, protein 22

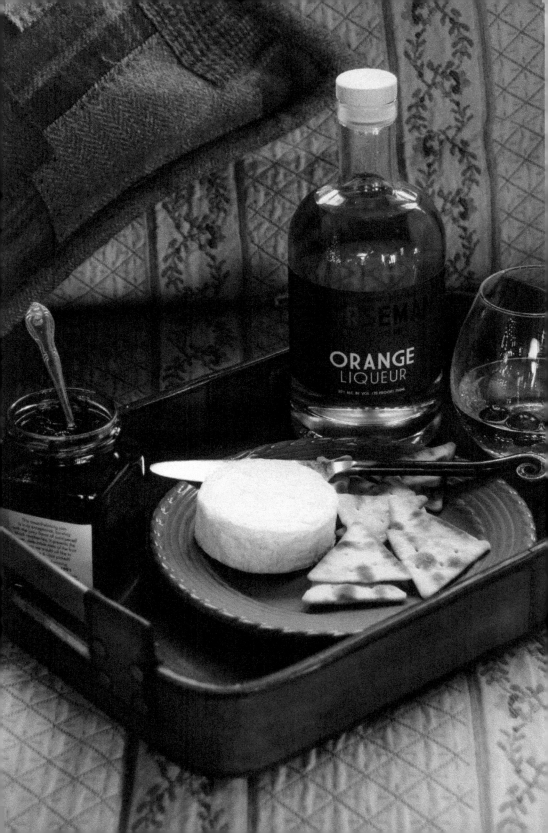

Conclusion

Here we come to the end of our keto cocktail journey. I hope that the keto cocktail recipes I have proposed to you have helped you improve your lifestyle. In addition to being tasty, these cocktails also have beneficial effects for the body. They help to combat different types of diseases and also to reduce your weight. I hope you will also recommend my book to your friends and family.

Good luck.

Lightning Source UK Ltd.
Milton Keynes UK
UKHW021833040621
384966UK00002B/481